# BREAST CANCER DIET COOKBOOK FOR WOMEN OVER 50

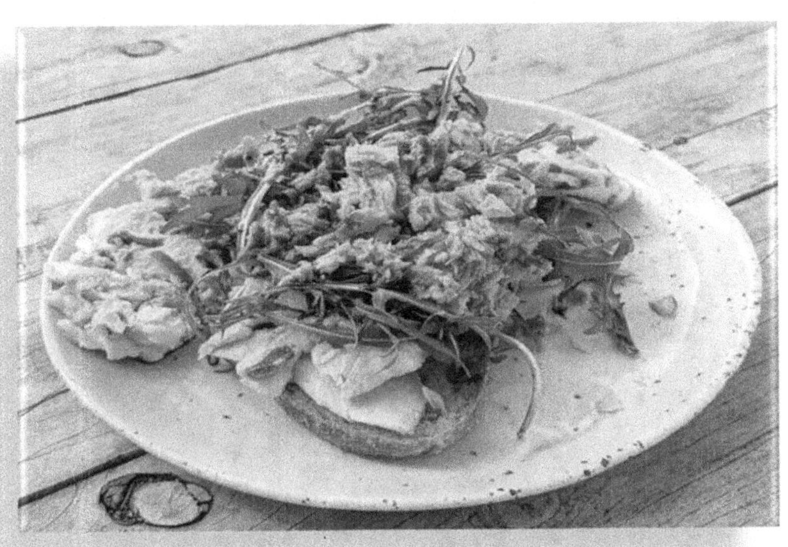

*The complete guide to healthy and delicious Anti-cancer researched plant-based recipes to heal the immune-system including 28 weeks meal plan for beginners.*

**CARLY EVELYN**

SCAN TO GET MORE BOOKS BY THIS AUTHOR

IF YOU ARE STUCK, WHILE PREPARING ANY RECIPES IN THIS COOKBOOK, YOU CAN REACH THE AUTHOR AT CARLYEVLCUISINEGUIDE@GMAIL.COM FOR GUIDANCE.........

# TABLE OF CONTENT

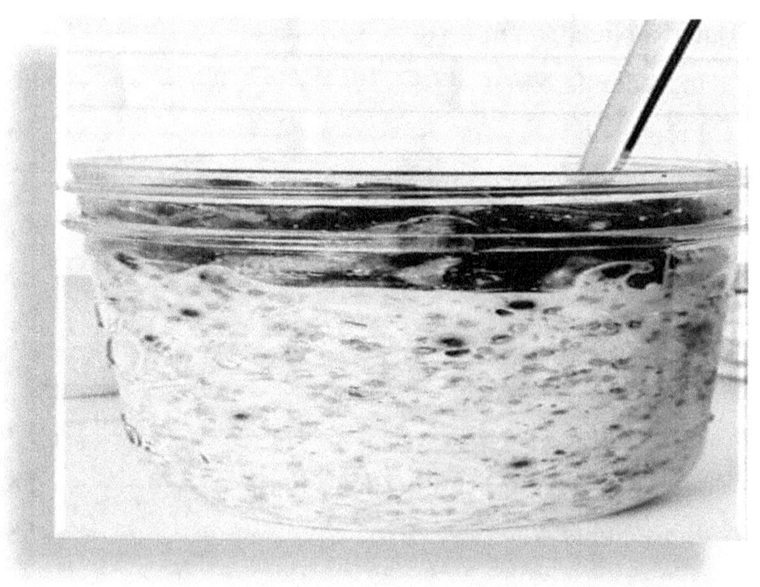

# INTRODUCTION

Once upon a time, in an artful senior community, lived Ms. Clara, a kind-hearted woman who was faced with the challenge of breast cancer. Undeterred, she discovered this magical cookbook called "Breast Cancer Diet Cookbook for Seniors."

With every turn of the page, Ms. Clara unraveled a world of nourishment and healing. This cookbook's recipes, thoughtfully crafted for seniors like her, were brimming with cancer-fighting ingredients that ignited hope within her heart. As she savored the flavors of vibrant fruits, vegetables, and wholesome grains, Ms. Clara noticed her energy surging, her body rejuvenating.

Amidst the warmth of family gatherings, Ms. Clara's culinary adventures became a joyous celebration of life and wellness. This cookbook's recipes fortified her spirit, bolstered her immune system, and instilled a newfound sense of empowerment. Supported by her loved ones and the cookbook's delicious fare, Ms. Clara found the strength to face her journey with courage and resilience.

In the end, Ms. Clara's story became an inspiring testament to the benefits of embracing a breast cancer diet tailored for seniors. This cookbook became her cherished ally, guiding her towards managing, controlling, and even reversing breast cancer. As she danced through life, her heart filled with gratitude, knowing that the power of nourishment and love had woven a miraculous tale of triumph.

## What is Breast Cancer

One of the most common cancers affecting women, although it can also occur in men, though much less frequently. Breast cancer is a type of cancer that begins in the cells of the breast. It occurs when abnormal cells in the breast grow and divide uncontrollably, forming a tumor.

## Breast Cancer and its Risk Factors

Breast cancer is a prevalent type of cancer that primarily affects women, although it can occur in men as well. It originates in the cells of the breast, potentially in various areas such as milk ducts or lobules, and it can manifest as either invasive or non-invasive forms.

## Common risk factors associated with breast cancer include

1. Gender: Women are at significantly higher risk compared to men.

2. Age: The likelihood of breast cancer increases with age, with most cases diagnosed in women over 50.

3. Family History: A family history of breast cancer can elevate one's risk.

4. Genetic Mutations: Inherited genetic mutations, such as those in the BRCA1 and BRCA2 genes, can substantially raise the risk.

5. Hormone-related Factors: Prolonged exposure to estrogen, through factors like early menstruation, late menopause, hormone replacement therapy, or specific contraceptives, can increase the risk.

6. Lifestyle Factors: Obesity, excessive alcohol consumption, and a sedentary lifestyle may contribute to an elevated risk.

Detecting breast cancer early is vital for effective treatment. Screening methods, such as mammograms, play a crucial role in early detection. Treatment options for breast cancer are diverse and may include surgery, radiation therapy, chemotherapy, hormone therapy, and targeted therapy.

## Types of Breast Cancer

Ductal Carcinoma in Situ (DCIS)- A non-invasive type of breast cancer where abnormal cells are found in the lining of a breast duct but haven't spread outside the duct.

Invasive Ductal Carcinoma (IDC)- The most common type of breast cancer, where cancer cells invade surrounding breast tissues.

Invasive Lobular Carcinoma (ILC)- This type of breast cancer begins in the milk-producing glands (lobules) and then invades nearby tissues.

Triple-Negative Breast Cancer- A subtype of breast cancer that lacks estrogen receptors, progesterone receptors, and HER2/neu protein, making it more difficult to treat with hormone-based therapies.

HER2-Positive Breast Cancer- A subtype of breast cancer where the cancer cells have an excess of a protein called human epidermal growth factor receptor 2 (HER2), promoting their growth.

## Symptoms of Breast Cancer

A bulge or thickening in the breast, underarm, or elsewhere.

Changes to the breast's size, shape, or appearance.

Unexplained pain in the breast or nipple.

Nipple discharge, especially if it is bloody and not breast milk.

Skin modifications, such as redness, dimpling, or scaling, on the breast.

## Preventive Measures for Breast Cancer

While some risk factors for breast cancer, such as age, gender, and family history, cannot be changed, there are several lifestyle changes and preventive measures that can help reduce the risk of breast cancer

Regular Breast Self-Exams- Perform monthly breast self-exams to become familiar with how your breasts normally look and feel, so you can promptly report any changes to your doctor.

Clinical Breast Exams- Have a clinical breast exam performed by a healthcare professional regularly, as recommended by your doctor.

Mammograms- Follow your doctor's recommendations for regular mammograms, which can help detect breast cancer early, even before symptoms are noticeable.

Maintain a Healthy Lifestyle- Adopt a healthy diet rich in fruits, vegetables, whole grains, and lean proteins. Maintain a healthy weight and partake in regular exercise.

Limit Alcohol Consumption- Limit or avoid alcohol consumption, as excessive alcohol intake has been linked to an increased risk of breast cancer.

Breastfeeding- If possible, breastfeed your babies, as it may have a protective effect against breast cancer.

Hormone Replacement- Therapy (HRT) If considering HRT to manage menopausal symptoms, discuss the potential risks and benefits with your healthcare provider, as long-term HRT use may slightly increase the risk of breast cancer.

Genetic Testing- If you have a strong family history of breast cancer or other risk factors, consider genetic counseling and testing to assess your individual risk.

Don't forget, while these measures can help reduce the risk of breast cancer, it's essential to discuss your specific situation with a healthcare professional to determine the best approach for your health. Regular check-ups and screenings are crucial for early detection and improved treatment outcomes.

While it's essential to maintain a healthy lifestyle and diet to help prevent or manage cancer A balanced diet rich in fruits, vegetables, whole grains, and lean proteins, along with regular exercise, can play a significant role in reducing the risk of cancer and promoting overall well-being.

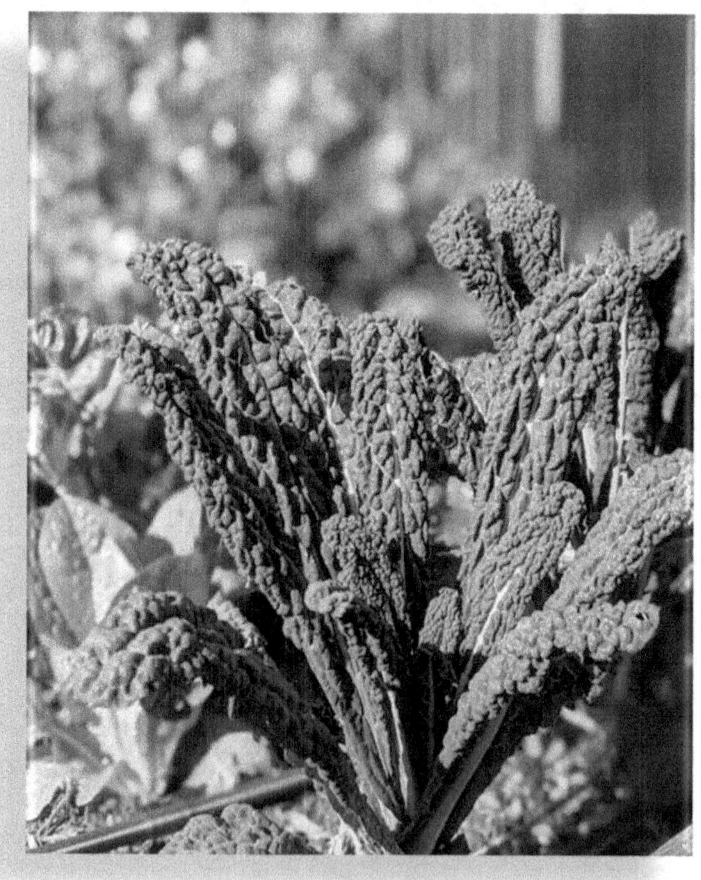

*Breakfast recipe that incorporate cancer-fighting ingredients and are generally considered healthy*

## Berry Breakfast Bowl

### Ingredients

Mixed berries (strawberries, blueberries, raspberries)
Greek yogurt (low-fat or non-fat)
Chia seeds
Honey or maple syrup (optional)

### Preparation

Combine the mixed berries and Greek yogurt in a bowl. Top with chia seeds and drizzle with honey or maple syrup for sweetness if desired.


## Avocado Toast

### Ingredients

Whole-grain bread
Avocado
Cherry tomatoes
Fresh basil leaves
Lemon juice
Salt and pepper to taste

### Preparation

Toast the whole-grain bread. Spread the avocado on the bread after mashing it. Top with sliced cherry tomatoes and fresh basil leaves. Season with salt and pepper and drizzle lemon juice on top.

## Spinach and Mushroom Omelette

### Ingredients

Eggs (2-3)
Baby spinach leaves
Button mushrooms, sliced
Onion, finely chopped
Garlic, minced
Olive oil
Salt and pepper to taste

### Preparation

In a skillet, heat olive oil and sauté the onions and garlic until fragrant. Add the sliced mushrooms and cook until tender. Add the baby spinach and let it wilt. Beat the eggs, season with salt and pepper, and pour over the vegetables in the skillet. Cook until the eggs are set, then fold the omelette and serve.

## Overnight Oats with Nuts and Seeds

### Ingredients

Rolled oats
Almond milk or any milk of choice
Chopped nuts (almonds, walnuts, etc.)
Ground flaxseeds
Fresh fruit (e.g., banana, apple, or berries)
Honey or maple syrup (optional)

*Preparation*

In a jar or bowl, mix the rolled oats, almond milk, chopped nuts, and ground flaxseeds. Cover and refrigerate overnight. In the morning, top with fresh fruit and drizzle with honey or maple syrup if desired.

## Quinoa Breakfast Bowl

### Ingredients

Cooked quinoa
Coconut milk or any milk of choice
Sliced bananas
Grated coconut
Chopped dates or raisins
Cinnamon powder

*Preparation*

In a bowl, mix cooked quinoa with coconut milk. Top with sliced bananas, grated coconut, chopped dates or raisins, and a sprinkle of cinnamon powder.

## Green Smoothie

### Ingredients

Spinach or kale
Banana
Green apple
Greek yogurt
Chia seeds
Water or almond milk

Blend spinach or kale with banana, green apple, Greek yogurt, chia seeds, and water or almond milk until smooth and creamy. When necessary, add extra liquid to change the consistency.

## Salmon and Avocado Wrap

### Ingredients

Whole-grain wrap or tortilla
Smoked salmon
Avocado slices
Cucumber slices
Mixed greens
Dill or parsley (optional)
Lemon juice
Salt and pepper to taste

### Preparation

Lay the whole-grain wrap on a flat surface. Layer smoked salmon, avocado slices, cucumber slices, and mixed greens. Sprinkle with dill or parsley if desired. Add salt and pepper, then drizzle with lemon juice. Roll the wrap and serve.

## Tomato and Basil Frittata

### Ingredients

Eggs (4-5)
Cherry tomatoes, halved
Fresh basil leaves
Garlic, minced
Olive oil
Salt and pepper to taste

Preheat the oven. In an oven-safe skillet, heat olive oil and sauté garlic until fragrant. After adding, sauté the cherry tomatoes until tender. Beat the eggs, season with salt and pepper, and pour over the tomatoes in the skillet. Arrange fresh basil leaves on top. Transfer the skillet to the oven and bake until the frittata is set and slightly golden.

## Blueberry and Almond Smoothie Bowl

### Ingredients

Frozen blueberries
Almond milk
Almond butter
Greek yogurt
Honey or maple syrup (optional)
Sliced almonds
Fresh blueberries

### Preparation

Blend frozen blueberries, almond milk, almond butter, Greek yogurt, and honey or maple syrup until smooth. Pour the smoothie into a bowl and top with sliced almonds and fresh blueberries.

## Chia Seed Pudding with Berries

### Ingredients

Chia seeds
Coconut milk or any milk of choice
Vanilla extract
Fresh berries (strawberries, blueberries, raspberries)
Honey or maple syrup (optional)

## Preparation

In a jar or bowl, mix chia seeds, coconut milk, and vanilla extract. Stir well and refrigerate for a few hours or overnight until the mixture thickens and forms a pudding-like consistency. Top with fresh berries and drizzle with honey or maple syrup if desired.

Remember to consult with a healthcare professional or registered dietitian for personalized dietary advice, especially if you are dealing with specific health conditions like cancer.

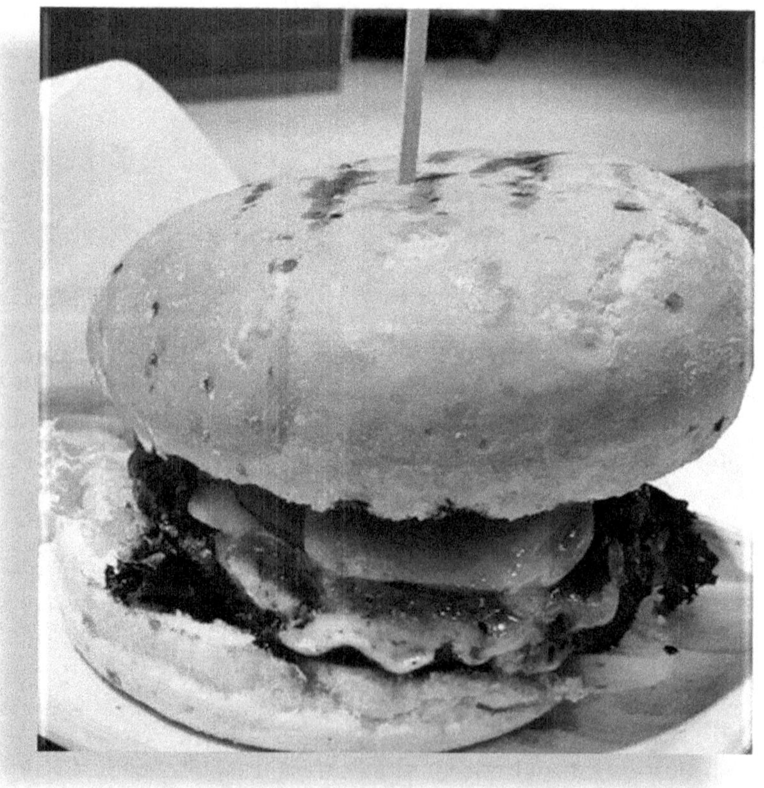

1. Incorporate an array of fresh fruits such as apples, berries, and citrus fruits.

2. Include a variety of fresh vegetables like leafy greens, carrots, and broccoli.

3. Opt for wholesome grains like brown rice and whole wheat bread.

4. Choose lean protein sources, such as chicken, turkey, and tofu.

5. Consider fatty fish like salmon, rich in omega-3 fatty acids.

6. Include eggs for protein and nutrients.

7. Select low-fat dairy products like yogurt and milk.

8. Add beans and legumes like lentils and chickpeas for fiber and protein.

9. Incorporate nuts and seeds like almonds and flaxseeds for healthy fats.

10. Opt for nut butter, such as almond butter.

11. Include oatmeal as a hearty and nutritious breakfast option.

12. Explore herbal teas like ginger and chamomile for soothing beverages.

13. Green tea is a fantastic choice for its potential health benefits.

14. Ginger is known to help alleviate nausea, which can be a side effect of treatment.

15. Turmeric, celebrated for its anti-inflammatory properties, can be used in cooking.

16. Use olive oil as a heart-healthy cooking oil.

17. Avocado is a nutritious and versatile addition to salads and dishes.

18. Incorporate quinoa for a high-protein, gluten-free grain.

19. Sweet potatoes provide a good source of vitamins and fiber.

20. Choose low-sugar, high-fiber cereal for breakfast options.

21. Low-sodium broth is useful for making nourishing homemade soups.

22. Elevate flavors with herbs and spices like basil and rosemary.

23. Sweeten dishes with honey or agave nectar as natural alternatives.

24. Unsweetened applesauce is a versatile ingredient in recipes.

25. Opt for canned fruits in natural juice to limit added sugars.

26. Stock up on smoothie ingredients like spinach and frozen fruits.

27. Greek yogurt is a protein-rich dairy product.

28. Enjoy cheese in moderation for added calcium.

29. Keep rice cakes on hand for a crunchy, low-calorie snack.

30. Hummus makes for a delicious and healthy dip.

31. Choose whole wheat pasta for a fiber-rich alternative.

32. Whole grain crackers provide a satisfying crunch.

33. Opt for low-sugar jam or preserves for a sweet touch.

34. Staying well-hydrated is crucial; drink plenty of water.

35. Consider coconut water as a natural electrolyte source.

36. Enjoy dark chocolate in moderation as a treat.

37. Pre-packaged protein shakes can be convenient for on-the-go nutrition.

38. Unsweetened almond milk is a dairy-free milk alternative.

39. Pre-cut and pre-washed vegetables offer convenience for quick meals.

40. Select low-sugar, high-protein snacks like protein bars for satisfying hunger.

Please note that the specific dietary needs of a breast cancer patient may differ based on their treatment and individual preferences

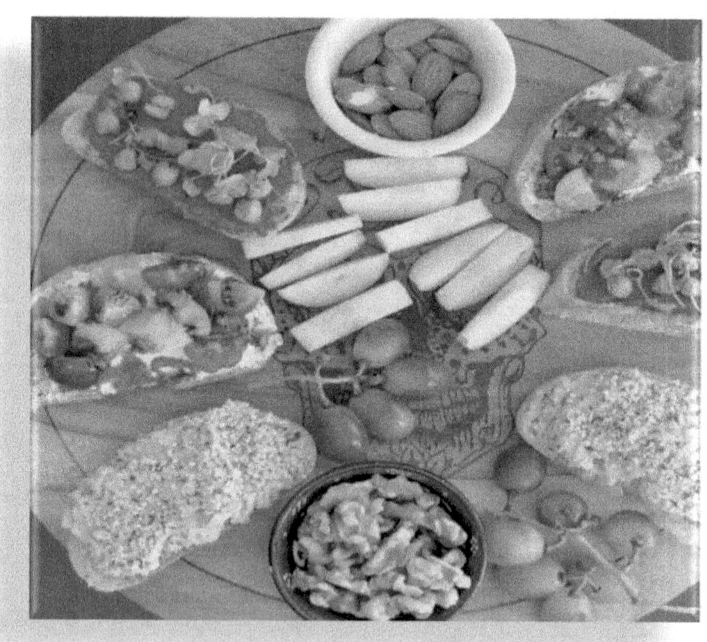

## Grilled Vegetable Salad

### Ingredients

Assorted vegetables (zucchini, bell peppers, eggplant, cherry
tomatoes, etc.)
Mixed salad greens (spinach, arugula, or kale)
Olive oil
Balsamic vinegar
Fresh basil or parsley
Salt and pepper to taste

### Preparation

Olive oil, salt, and pepper should be added to the veggies.
 Grill them until they are lightly charred and tender. Arrange
the grilled vegetables over a bed of mixed salad greens.
Drizzle with balsamic vinegar and garnish with fresh basil
or parsley.

## Lentil and Kale Soup

### Ingredients

Green or brown lentils
Kale, chopped
Carrots, diced
Celery, diced
Onion, chopped
Garlic, minced
Vegetable broth
Olive oil

Turmeric powder
Salt and pepper to taste


### Preparation

In a large pot, heat olive oil and sauté onions and garlic until fragrant. Add the diced carrots and celery and cook until softened. Rinse the lentils and add them to the pot along with vegetable broth. Bring to a boil, then reduce heat and simmer until lentils are cooked. Stir in chopped kale, turmeric powder, salt, and pepper. The kale should be soft after a few more minutes of simmering.

## Quinoa and Broccoli Stir-Fry

### Ingredients

Cooked quinoa
Broccoli florets
Red bell pepper, sliced
Carrots, julienned
Scallions, chopped
Soy sauce (low-sodium)
Sesame oil
Garlic, minced
Ginger, grated
Sesame seeds (optional)

### Preparation

In a wok or large skillet, heat sesame oil and sauté garlic and ginger until fragrant. Include the carrots, red bell pepper, and broccoli. Stir-fry until the vegetables are tender-crisp. Add cooked quinoa and scallions to the pan, and drizzle with soy sauce. Toss everything together until well combined. Sprinkle with sesame seeds if desired.

## Baked Salmon with Lemon and Dill

### Ingredients

Salmon fillet
Lemon slices
Fresh dill
Olive oil
Garlic, minced
Salt and pepper to taste

### Preparation

Preheat the oven. Place the salmon fillet on a baking sheet lined with parchment paper. Drizzle with olive oil and sprinkle minced garlic, salt, and pepper over the fish. Top with lemon slices and fresh dill. Salmon should be baked in the oven until it is well done and flakes with a fork with ease.

## Chickpea and Cucumber Salad

### Ingredients

Cooked chickpeas
Cucumber, diced
Cherry tomatoes, halved
Red onion, thinly sliced
Fresh parsley or cilantro
Lemon juice
Olive oil
Ground cumin
Salt and pepper to taste

### Preparation

In a bowl, combine chickpeas, diced cucumber, halved cherry tomatoes, and sliced red onion. Drizzle with lemon juice and olive oil. Sprinkle ground cumin, salt, and pepper over the salad. Toss gently to combine and garnish with fresh parsley or cilantro.

## Brown Rice Sushi Rolls

### Ingredients

Nori seaweed sheets
Cooked brown rice
Avocado slices
Cucumber strips
Carrot strips
Cooked shrimp or smoked salmon (optional)
Low-sodium soy sauce or tamari

### Preparation

Lay a nori sheet on a bamboo sushi rolling mat. Spread a layer of cooked brown rice over the nori, leaving a small border at the top. Place avocado slices, cucumber strips, and carrot strips along the center of the rice. Add cooked shrimp or smoked salmon if desired. Roll the sushi tightly using the bamboo mat. To seal the roll, wet the top border with water. Slice the sushi roll into bite-sized pieces and serve with low-sodium soy sauce or tamari.

## Tofu and Vegetable Stir-Fry

### Ingredients

Firm tofu, cubed
Assorted vegetables (bell peppers, broccoli, snap peas, etc.)
Garlic, minced
Ginger, grated
Low-sodium soy sauce or tamari
Sesame oil

Green onions, sliced
Sesame seeds (optional)

## Preparation

In a wok or large skillet, heat sesame oil and sauté minced garlic and grated ginger until fragrant. Stir-fry the tofu cubes until they are just beginning to color. Add the assorted vegetables and continue stir-frying until they are tender-crisp. Drizzle with low-sodium soy sauce or tamari and toss to coat. If desired, garnish with sesame seeds and thinly sliced green onions.

# Whole Grain Pasta with Tomato and Basil

## Ingredients

Whole grain pasta
Cherry tomatoes, halved
Fresh basil leaves
Garlic, minced
Olive oil
Balsamic vinegar
Salt and pepper to taste

## Preparation

Follow the directions on the package to prepare the whole-grain pasta. Garlic cloves that have been minced should be cooked in olive oil until aromatic.
Add halved cherry tomatoes and cook until softened. Combine the tomato mixture with the cooked pasta. Drizzle with balsamic vinegar, sprinkle with torn fresh basil leaves, and season with salt and pepper.

## Rainbow Quinoa Salad

### Ingredients

Cooked rainbow quinoa
Mixed bell peppers, diced
Shredded purple cabbage
Shredded carrots
Sliced radishes
Fresh cilantro or parsley
Lemon juice
Olive oil
Honey or maple syrup (optional)
Salt and pepper to taste

### Preparation

In a large bowl, combine cooked rainbow quinoa, diced mixed bell peppers, shredded purple cabbage, shredded carrots, and sliced radishes. Drizzle with lemon juice and olive oil. If you want more sweetness, you may add honey or maple syrup. Toss everything together until well combined. Garnish with fresh cilantro or parsley.

## Stuffed Bell Peppers with Quinoa and Beans

### Ingredients

Bell peppers (assorted colors)
Cooked quinoa
Cooked black beans or kidney beans
Diced tomatoes
Onion, chopped
Garlic, minced
Ground cumin

Paprika
Salt and pepper to taste
Grated cheese (optional)

## *Preparation*

Preheat the oven. Remove the bell peppers' tops, then scoop out the seeds and membranes. In a skillet, sauté chopped onions and minced garlic until softened. Add diced tomatoes, cooked quinoa, cooked black beans or kidney beans, ground cumin, paprika, salt, and pepper. Cook until heated through. Stuff the bell peppers with the quinoa and bean mixture. If desired, top with grated cheese. The filled peppers should be placed on a baking tray and baked in the oven until the cheese has melted and the peppers are soft.

These lunch recipes incorporate a variety of cancer-fighting ingredients and provide a nutritious and delicious meal

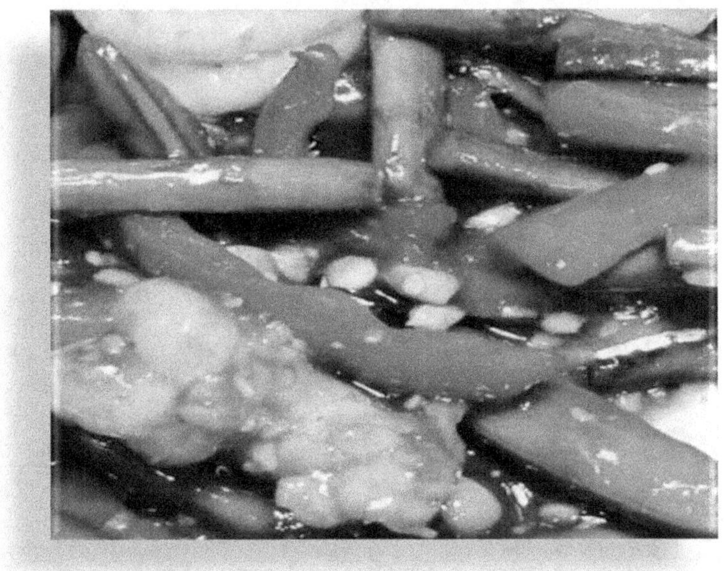

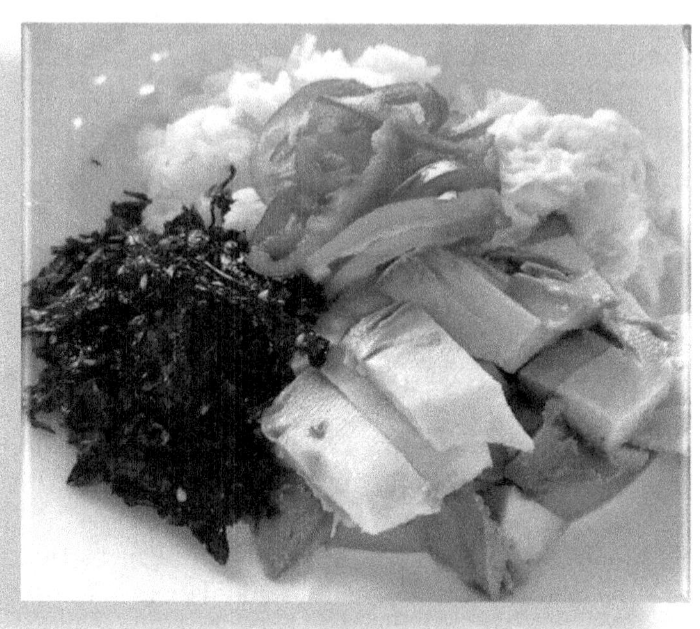

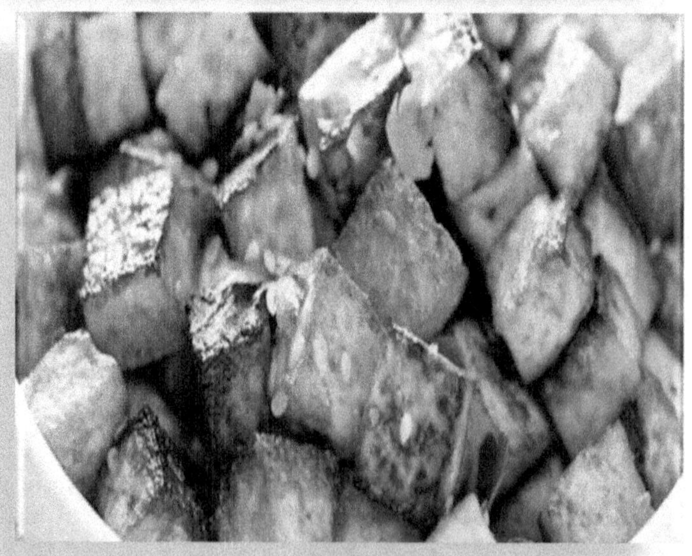

1. **Maintain a Healthy Weight**: Strive to keep a healthy weight since excess weight, especially after menopause, is associated with an increased risk of breast cancer.

2. **Regular Physical Activity**: Incorporate at least 150 minutes of moderate-intensity exercise weekly, such as brisk walking, to decrease your risk.

3. **Limit Alcohol**: Exercise caution with alcohol consumption, as excessive drinking has a known association with an elevated risk of breast cancer.

4. **Healthy Diet**: Embrace a well-rounded diet replete with fruits, vegetables, whole grains, and lean proteins.

5. **Breastfeed**: If you're able, consider breastfeeding your children, as it can potentially reduce your risk of breast cancer.

6. **Hormone Replacement Therapy**: Be discerning about hormone replacement therapy, as it can heighten the risk in certain women. Consult your healthcare provider to explore suitable options.

7. **Regular Self-Exams**: Cultivate a monthly habit of self-examining your breasts to become intimately acquainted with them and promptly detect any changes.

8. **Clinical Breast Exams**: Prioritize regular clinical breast exams conducted by your healthcare provider.

9.   **Mammograms**: Abide by the recommended mammogram guidelines tailored to your age and specific risk factors.

10. **Know Your Family History**: Acquaint yourself with your family's breast cancer history and transparently communicate this information with your healthcare provider.

11. **Genetic Counseling**: If a family history of breast cancer exists, contemplate genetic counseling to evaluate your individual risk.

12. **Avoid Exposure to Environmental Toxins**: Be mindful of environmental toxins, such as pesticides and industrial chemicals, and take steps to minimize exposure.

13. **Healthy Fats**: Opt for healthful fats found in sources like olive oil and avocados while curbing intake of saturated and trans fats.

14. **Limit Sugar Intake**: Diminish the presence of added sugars in your diet, a step that may contribute to lowering your cancer risk.

15. **Quit Smoking**: If you smoke, seek professional support to quit, as smoking is correlated with several cancer types.

16. **Sun Protection**: Shield your skin from harmful UV radiation, as excess sun exposure can heighten the breast cancer risk.

17. **Limit Radiation Exposure**: Exercise prudence to restrict unnecessary exposure to radiation, particularly during medical procedures.

18. **Manage Stress**: Prioritize stress management techniques, including practices like meditation and yoga, as chronic stress can adversely impact your well-being.

19. **Early Detection**: Attend regular medical check-ups and screening appointments, which encompass vital procedures like mammograms, enabling early breast cancer detection.

20. **Stay Informed**: Stay well-informed about breast cancer risk factors and prevention strategies, allowing you to make informed choices that safeguard your health.

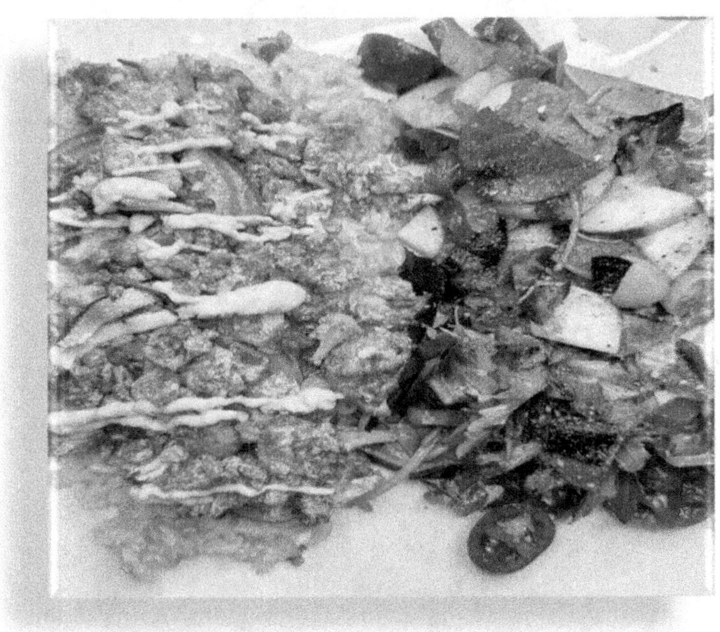

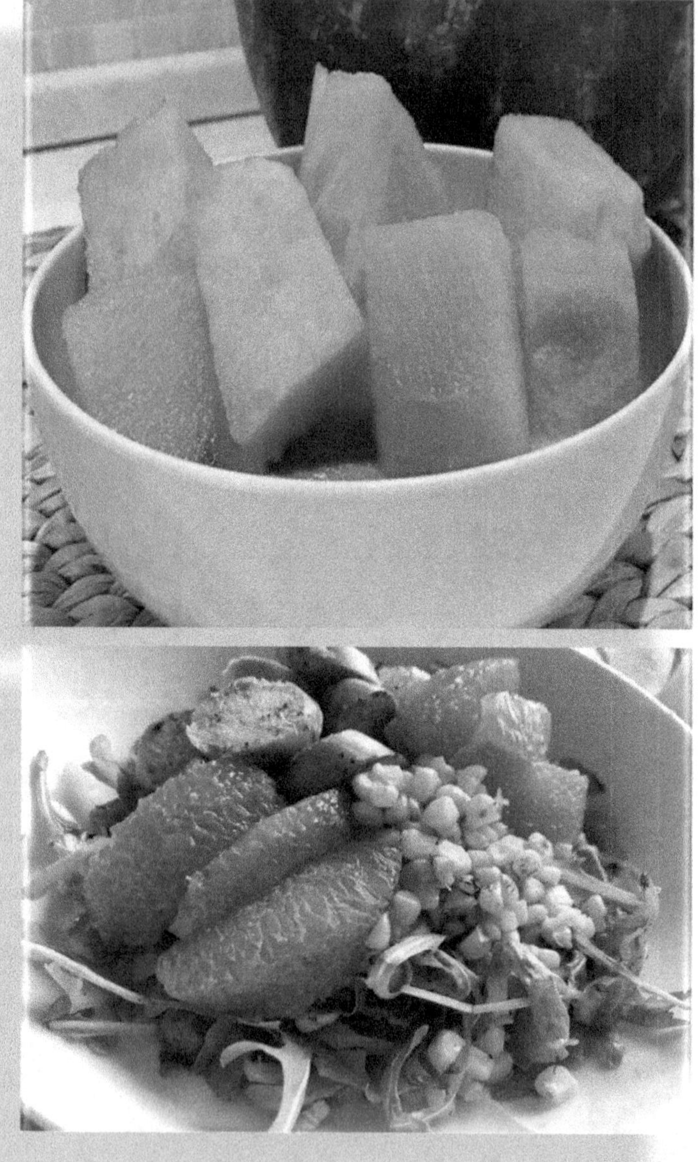

## Grilled Lemon Herb Chicken

### Ingredients

Boneless, skinless chicken breasts
Lemon juice
Fresh thyme or rosemary
Garlic, minced
Olive oil
Salt and pepper to taste

### Preparation

In a bowl, mix lemon juice, minced garlic, chopped fresh thyme or rosemary, olive oil, salt, and pepper to create a marinade. Put the marinade over the chicken breasts and let them sit for at least 30 minutes. Grill the chicken until cooked through and slightly charred.

## Roasted Vegetable Quinoa Bowl

### Ingredients

Assorted vegetables (sweet potatoes, Brussels sprouts, cauliflower, etc.)
Olive oil
Cooked quinoa
Chickpeas (optional)
Lemon tahini dressing (lemon juice, tahini, garlic, water, salt)

Preheat the oven. Toss the assorted vegetables with olive oil, salt, and pepper. The veggies should be baked until they are soft and caramelized. In a bowl, layer the roasted vegetables, cooked quinoa, and chickpeas (if using). Drizzle with lemon tahini dressing.

## Broiled Salmon with Garlic and Herbs

### Ingredients

Salmon fillet
Garlic, minced
Fresh dill or parsley
Lemon zest
Olive oil
Salt and pepper to taste

### Preparation

Preheat the broiler. Place the salmon fillet on a baking sheet lined with parchment paper. Mix minced garlic, chopped dill or parsley, lemon zest, olive oil, salt, and pepper to create a paste. Spread the paste over the salmon. Broil the salmon in the oven until it's cooked through and lightly browned on top.

## Veggie Stir-Fry with Tofu

### Ingredients

Firm tofu, cubed
Various veggies, including broccoli, bell peppers, and snap peas
Low-sodium soy sauce or tamari
Sesame oil

Ginger, grated
Garlic, minced
Green onions, sliced
Sesame seeds (optional)

*Preparation*

In a wok or large skillet, heat sesame oil and sauté grated ginger and minced garlic until fragrant. Add cubed tofu and stir-fry until lightly browned. Add the assorted vegetables and continue stir-frying until they are tender-crisp. Drizzle with low-sodium soy sauce or tamari and toss to coat. If desired, garnish with sesame seeds and thinly sliced green onions.

## Whole Grain Spaghetti with Tomato Basil Sauce

*Ingredients*

Whole grain spaghetti
Fresh tomatoes, diced
Fresh basil leaves
Garlic, minced
Olive oil
Balsamic vinegar
Salt and pepper to taste

*Preparation*

Cook the whole grain spaghetti according to the package instructions. In a separate pan, sauté minced garlic in olive oil until fragrant. Add diced fresh tomatoes and cook until softened. Toss the cooked spaghetti with the tomato mixture. Drizzle with balsamic vinegar, tear fresh basil leaves over the top, and season with salt and pepper.

## Grilled Shrimp and Vegetable Skewers

### Ingredients

Shrimp, peeled and deveined
various veggies (such as cherry tomatoes, zucchini, and bell peppers)
Olive oil
Lemon juice
Garlic, minced
Fresh parsley or cilantro
Salt and pepper to taste

### Preparation

Preheat the grill. Thread the shrimp and assorted vegetables onto skewers. Mix olive oil, lemon juice, minced garlic, chopped parsley or cilantro, salt, and pepper to create a marinade. Brush the skewers with the marinade. Grill the skewers until the shrimp are cooked through and the vegetables are tender and slightly charred.

## Lentil and Vegetable Curry

### Ingredients

Green or brown lentils
Mixed vegetables (carrots, bell peppers, cauliflower, etc.)
Onion, chopped
Garlic, minced
Ginger, grated
Curry powder
Coconut milk
Vegetable broth
Olive oil
Fresh cilantro (optional)

Cooked brown rice or quinoa (for serving)

*Preparation*

In a large pot, heat olive oil and sauté chopped onions, minced garlic, and grated ginger until fragrant. Add mixed vegetables and cook until they are slightly softened. Lentils should be rinsed before adding to the saucepan. Add the coconut milk, vegetable broth, and curry powder. Bring to a boil, then reduce heat and simmer until the lentils are cooked and the curry has thickened. Serve over cooked brown rice or quinoa and garnish with fresh cilantro if desired.

## Stuffed Bell Peppers with Quinoa and Lentils

### Ingredients

Bell peppers (assorted colors)
Cooked quinoa
Cooked green or brown lentils
Diced tomatoes
Onion, chopped
Garlic, minced
Fresh thyme or rosemary
Salt and pepper to taste
Grated cheese (optional)

### Preparation

Preheat the oven. Remove the bell peppers' tops, then scoop out the seeds and membranes. In a skillet, sauté chopped onions and minced garlic until softened. Add diced tomatoes, cooked quinoa, cooked lentils, chopped fresh thyme or rosemary, salt, and pepper. Cook until heated through. Stuff the bell peppers with the quinoa and lentil mixture. If desired, top with grated cheese. The filled peppers should be placed on a baking tray and baked in the oven until the cheese has melted and the peppers are soft.

## Baked Sweet Potato with Black Bean and Avocado Salsa

### Ingredients

Sweet potatoes
Black beans, drained and rinsed
Avocado, diced
Cherry tomatoes, halved
Red onion, finely chopped
Fresh cilantro
Lime juice
Olive oil
Salt and pepper to taste

### Preparation

Preheat the oven. Pierce the sweet potatoes with a fork and bake them in the oven until tender. In a bowl, mix black beans, diced avocado, halved cherry tomatoes, finely chopped red onion, and chopped cilantro. Add lime juice, olive oil, salt, and pepper to the dressing. Cut open the baked sweet potatoes and stuff with the black bean and avocado salsa.

# Grilled Vegetable and Chickpea Salad

## Ingredients

Assorted vegetables (asparagus, eggplant, red onion, etc.)
Chickpeas
Fresh basil or parsley
Lemon juice
Olive oil
Balsamic vinegar
Salt and pepper to taste

## Preparation

Toss the assorted vegetables and chickpeas in olive oil, salt, and pepper. Grill the vegetables and chickpeas until they are lightly charred and tender. In a bowl, combine the grilled vegetables and chickpeas. Drizzle with lemon juice and balsamic vinegar. Garnish with fresh basil or parsley.

These dinner recipes aim to provide a variety of cancer-fighting nutrients and delicious flavors

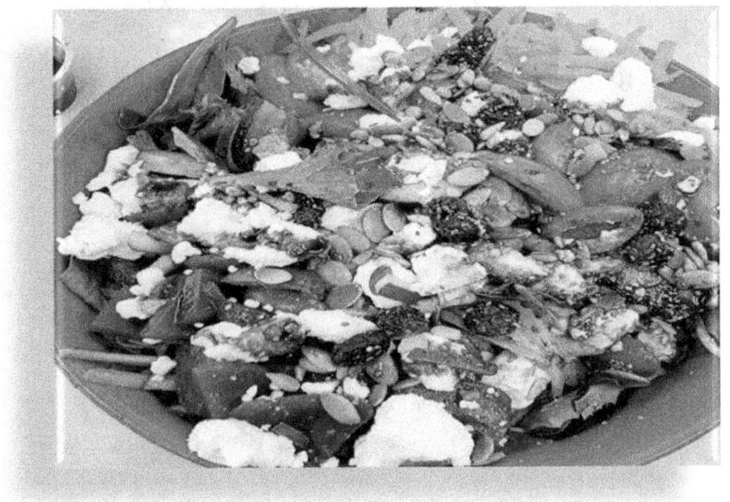

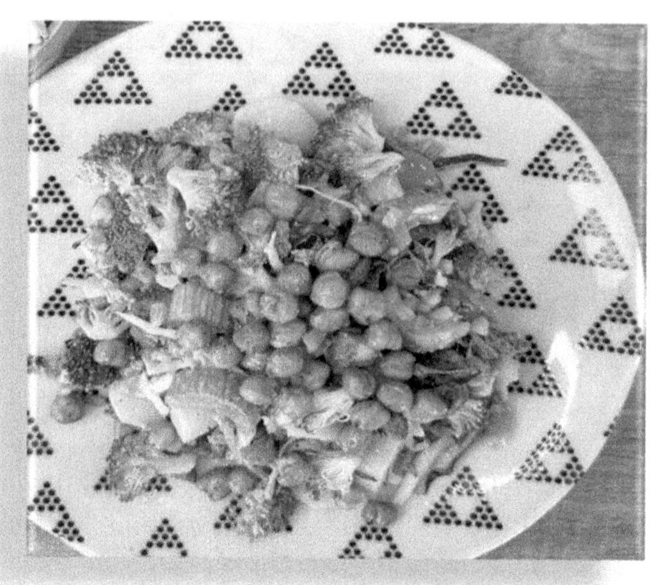

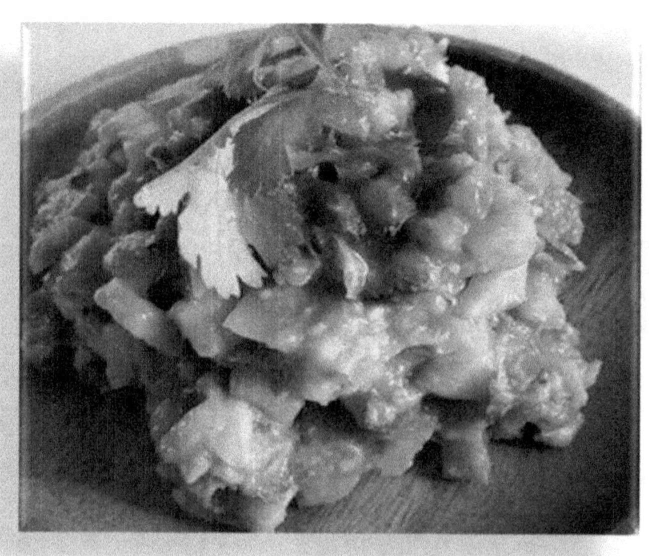

*Healthy and tasty snack recipes an excellent opportunity to incorporate cancer-fighting ingredients into your diet*

## Hummus with Vegetable Sticks

### Ingredients

Chickpeas (canned or cooked)
Tahini
Lemon juice
Garlic, minced
Olive oil
Salt and pepper to taste
Assorted vegetable sticks (carrots, cucumber, bell peppers)

### Preparation

In a food processor, blend chickpeas, tahini, lemon juice, minced garlic, olive oil, salt, and pepper until smooth. Serve with assorted vegetable sticks for dipping.

## Greek Yogurt Parfait

### Ingredients

Greek yogurt (low-fat or non-fat)
Fresh berries (strawberries, blueberries, raspberries)
Honey or maple syrup
Granola or chopped nuts (almonds, walnuts)

### Preparation

In a glass or bowl, layer Greek yogurt, fresh berries, and drizzle with honey or maple syrup. Top with granola or chopped nuts for added crunch.

# Guacamole with Whole Grain Pita Chips

## Ingredients

Ripe avocados
Diced tomatoes
Diced red onion
Fresh cilantro
Lime juice
Salt and pepper to taste
Whole grain pita bread, cut into triangles

## Preparation

In a bowl, mash ripe avocados and mix with diced tomatoes, diced red onion, chopped cilantro, lime juice, salt, and pepper. Serve with whole grain pita chips for dipping.

# Edamame Salad

## Ingredients

Cooked edamame (soybeans)
Cherry tomatoes, halved
Diced cucumber
Sliced radishes
Chopped fresh mint or basil
Lemon juice
Olive oil
Salt and pepper to taste

## Preparation

In a bowl, combine cooked edamame, halved cherry tomatoes, diced cucumber, sliced radishes, and chopped fresh mint or basil. Add lemon juice, olive oil, salt, and pepper to the dressing

## Baked Kale Chips

### Ingredients

Fresh kale leaves
Olive oil
Salt and pepper to taste

### Preparation

Preheat the oven. Remove the stems from the kale leaves and tear them into bite-sized pieces. Toss the kale pieces with olive oil, salt, and pepper. Spread the kale on a baking sheet in a single layer. Bake in the oven until the kale is crispy but not burnt.

## Almond Butter and Banana Toast

### Ingredients

Whole-grain bread
Almond butter
Sliced banana
Chia seeds (optional)
Honey (optional)

### Preparation

Toast the whole-grain bread. Toast should be spread with almond butter, then topped with banana slices.
 Sprinkle with chia seeds and drizzle with honey for added sweetness if desired.

## Turmeric Roasted Chickpeas

### Ingredients

Chickpeas (canned or cooked)
Olive oil
Ground turmeric
Ground cumin
Ground coriander
Salt and pepper to taste

### Preparation

Preheat the oven. Pat dries the chickpeas and toss them with olive oil, ground turmeric, ground cumin, ground coriander, salt, and pepper. Spread the chickpeas on a baking sheet in a single layer. Bake in the oven until the chickpeas are crispy.


## Carrot and Beetroot Slaw

### Ingredients

Carrots, grated
Beetroot, grated
Fresh parsley or cilantro
Lemon juice
Olive oil
Honey or maple syrup (optional)
Chopped walnuts (optional)

### Preparation

In a bowl, combine grated carrots, grated beetroot, chopped parsley or cilantro. Dress with lemon juice, olive oil, and honey or maple syrup if desired for sweetness. For more crunch, sprinkle chopped walnuts on top.

## Smoked Salmon Cucumber Bites

### Ingredients

Cucumber, sliced into rounds
Smoked salmon slices
Greek yogurt (low-fat or non-fat)
Fresh dill or chives

### Preparation

Top each cucumber round with a slice of smoked salmon. Add a small dollop of Greek yogurt on top. Garnish with fresh dill or chives.

## Berry and Spinach Smoothie

### Ingredients

Fresh spinach
Mixed berries (strawberries, blueberries, raspberries)
Banana
Greek yogurt (low-fat or non-fat)
Chia seeds
Water or almond milk

### Preparation

Blend fresh spinach, mixed berries, banana, Greek yogurt, chia seeds, and water or almond milk until smooth and creamy.

These snack recipes provide a combination of cancer-fighting ingredients, nutrients, and flavors. Remember to enjoy snacks in moderation as part of a balanced diet. If you have specific dietary restrictions or health concerns, it's best to consult with a healthcare professional or registered dietitian for personalized advice.

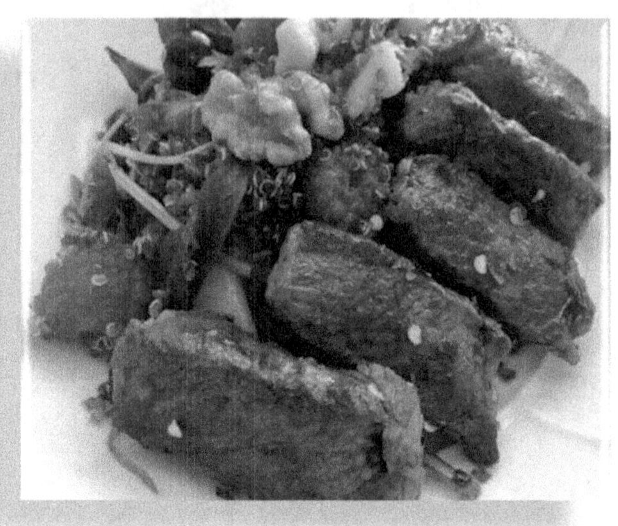

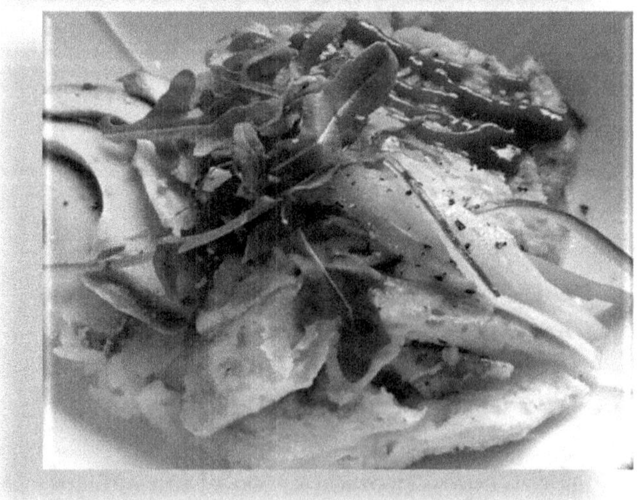

1. Arm Circles:
   - Position your feet shoulder-width apart.
   - Extend your arms outward to the sides.
   - Commence making small circles with your arms, gradually expanding the diameter.

2. Wall Push-Ups:
   - Face a wall.
   - Place your hands flat on the wall, aligned with your shoulders.
   - Proceed to bend your elbows, drawing your chest nearer to the wall, and then gently push back.

3. Chair Squats:
   - Sit on a sturdy chair, feet hip-width apart.
   - Transition from a seated position to a standing one, but do not fully sit down again, mimicking the motion of sitting.

4. Seated Leg Lifts:
   - Sit in a chair, ensuring your feet rest flat on the floor.
   - Elevate one leg straight out and sustain the position momentarily, then lower it.
   - Cycle between legs.

5. Shoulder Blade Squeezes:

- Be seated or stand, maintaining an upright posture.
    - Consciously squeeze your shoulder blades together for a few seconds, then release.

6. Side Leg Lifts:
    - Take a position with one hand for stability.
    - Elevate one leg sideways and then lower it.
    - Perform this exercise on the opposite side.

7. Chest Opener Stretch:
    - Stand with feet hip-width apart.
    - Clasp your hands behind your back and gently draw your arms back to open up your chest.

8. March in Place:
    - Engage in a few minutes of marching in place, lifting your knees high to enhance cardiovascular fitness.

9. Ankle Circles:
    - Sit in a chair, feet grounded.
    - Elevate one leg and execute circular motions with your ankle.
    - Repeat the process with the other leg.

10. Neck Tilts:
    - Maintain an upright position in a chair.
    - Tilt your head gently to one side, bringing your ear nearer to your shoulder, maintaining the tilt for a few seconds.
    - Replicate this motion on the opposite side.


11. Bicep Curls:

- Secure a lightweight object (e.g., a water bottle) in each hand.
- With palms facing forward, perform bicep curls by raising the weights towards your shoulders.

12. Hip Circles:
- Position your feet hip-width apart.
- Execute circular movements with your hips, beginning with clockwise rotations and subsequently counterclockwise.

13. Stair Climbing:
- When accessible, ascend and descend stairs to enhance leg strength and cardiovascular fitness.

14. Calf Raises:
- Stand with feet hip-width apart.
- Raise onto your toes, and then gently lower your heels back to the ground.

15. Seated Row:
- Be seated on a sturdy chair, ensuring your feet rest flat.
- Secure a resistance band or towel with both hands, and draw it towards your chest, retracting your shoulder blades together.

16. Knee Extensions:
- Be seated in a chair with feet grounded flat on the floor.
- Extend one leg straight and uphold the position for a brief duration.
- Rotate between legs.

17. Chest Press:

- Take a seat on a chair or bench, feet grounded flat.
   - Hold a lightweight in each hand and propel your arms forward.

18. Triceps Dips:
   - Position yourself on the edge of a robust chair or bench, hands situated beside your hips.
   - Elevation of your body off the chair and then descent.

19. Toe Taps:
   - Be seated in a chair and rhythmically tap your toes on the floor or a small step situated in front of you.

20. Back Leg Raises:
   - Stand with your hands resting on a stable surface.
   - Elevate one leg backward and then gently lower it.
   - Recur the procedure on the opposite side.

It is imperative to embark on these exercises gradually, adhering to your comfort level, and incrementally intensify the duration or intensity as your strength and endurance progress.

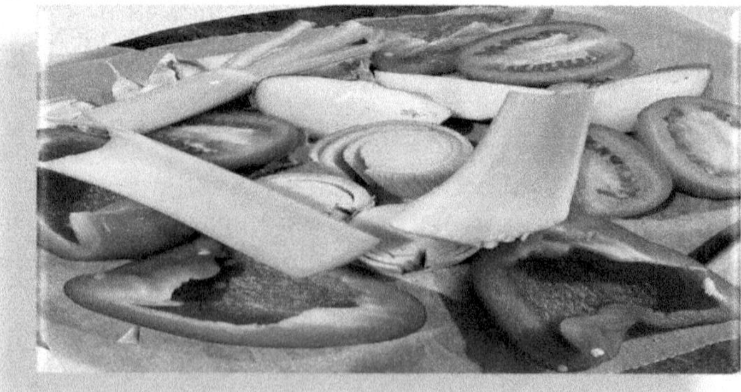

## Mixed Berry Chia Seed Pudding

### Ingredients

Mixed berries (strawberries, blueberries, raspberries)
Chia seeds
Almond milk or any milk of choice
Honey or maple syrup (optional)

### Preparation

In a jar or bowl, mix chia seeds and almond milk. Add a handful of mixed berries and stir well. Cover and refrigerate overnight or for a few hours until the mixture thickens and forms a pudding-like consistency. If desired, drizzle with honey or maple syrup for added sweetness.

## Dark Chocolate Dipped Strawberries

### Ingredients

Fresh strawberries
Dark chocolate (at least 70% cocoa)

### Preparation

Melt the dark chocolate in a double boiler or microwave. Dip the strawberries into the melted chocolate and place them on a parchment-lined tray. Refrigerate until the chocolate hardens.

# Baked Apples with Cinnamon and Almonds

## Ingredients

Apples (such as Granny Smith or Honeycrisp)
Ground cinnamon
Chopped almonds
Honey (optional)

## Preparation

Preheat the oven. Core the apples and place them in a baking dish. Sprinkle ground cinnamon and chopped almonds over the apples. If desired, drizzle with honey. Bake in the oven until the apples are soft and tender.

# Banana Nice Cream

## Ingredients

Ripe bananas, sliced and frozen
Almond milk or any milk of choice
Peanut butter (optional)
Dark chocolate chips (optional)

## Preparation

In a blender or food processor, blend frozen banana slices with almond milk until creamy and smooth. For added flavor, mix in a spoonful of peanut butter or sprinkle in some dark chocolate chips.

# Avocado Chocolate Mousse

## Ingredients

Ripe avocados
Unsweetened cocoa powder
Almond milk or any milk of choice
Honey or maple syrup (optional)
Fresh berries (for topping)

## Preparation

In a blender or food processor, blend ripe avocados, unsweetened cocoa powder, and almond milk until smooth and creamy. Add honey or maple syrup for sweetness if desired. Serve the chocolate mousse with fresh berries on top.


# Oatmeal Raisin Cookies

## Ingredients

Rolled oats
Whole wheat flour
Raisins
Coconut oil or unsalted butter
Honey or maple syrup
Eggs (or flaxseed mixture for egg replacement)
Ground cinnamon
Baking soda
Salt

## Preparation

Preheat the oven. In a bowl, mix rolled oats, whole wheat flour, raisins, melted coconut oil or unsalted butter, honey or maple syrup, eggs (or flaxseed mixture), ground cinnamon, baking soda, and salt. Form the dough into cookie shapes on a baking sheet lined with parchment paper. Bake in the oven until the cookies are golden brown.

## Yogurt and Mixed Fruit Parfait

### Ingredients

Greek yogurt (low-fat or non-fat)
Mixed fruits (such as berries, kiwi, and mango)
Granola or chopped nuts (optional)
Honey or maple syrup (optional)

### Preparation

In a glass or bowl, layer Greek yogurt with mixed fruits. If desired, add granola or chopped nuts for added crunch. Drizzle with honey or maple syrup for sweetness.

## Pumpkin Spice Energy Bites

### Ingredients

Rolled oats
Pumpkin puree
Almond butter
Ground cinnamon
Ground nutmeg
Honey or maple syrup
Chia seeds

### Preparation

In a bowl, mix rolled oats, pumpkin puree, almond butter, ground cinnamon, ground nutmeg, honey or maple syrup, and chia seeds. Make bite-sized balls out of the mixture and chill until hard.

## Berry and Almond Crisp

### Ingredients

Mixed berries (strawberries, blueberries, raspberries)
Almond flour
Rolled oats
Chopped almonds
Coconut oil or unsalted butter
Honey or maple syrup

### Preparation

Preheat the oven. In a baking dish, place mixed berries. In a separate bowl, mix almond flour, rolled oats, chopped almonds, melted coconut oil or unsalted butter, and honey or maple syrup. Spread the crumble mixture over the berries. Bake in the oven until the berries are bubbling and the topping is golden brown.

## Watermelon and Mint Sorbet

### Ingredients

Fresh watermelon, cubed and frozen
Fresh mint leaves
Lime juice
Honey or maple syrup (optional)

### Preparation

In a blender or food processor, blend frozen watermelon cubes with fresh mint leaves and lime juice until smooth and slushy. If desired, sweeten with honey or maple syrup.

These dessert recipes offer a healthier twist on classic favorites and incorporate cancer-fighting ingredients. As with any treat, enjoy them in moderation as part of a balanced diet.

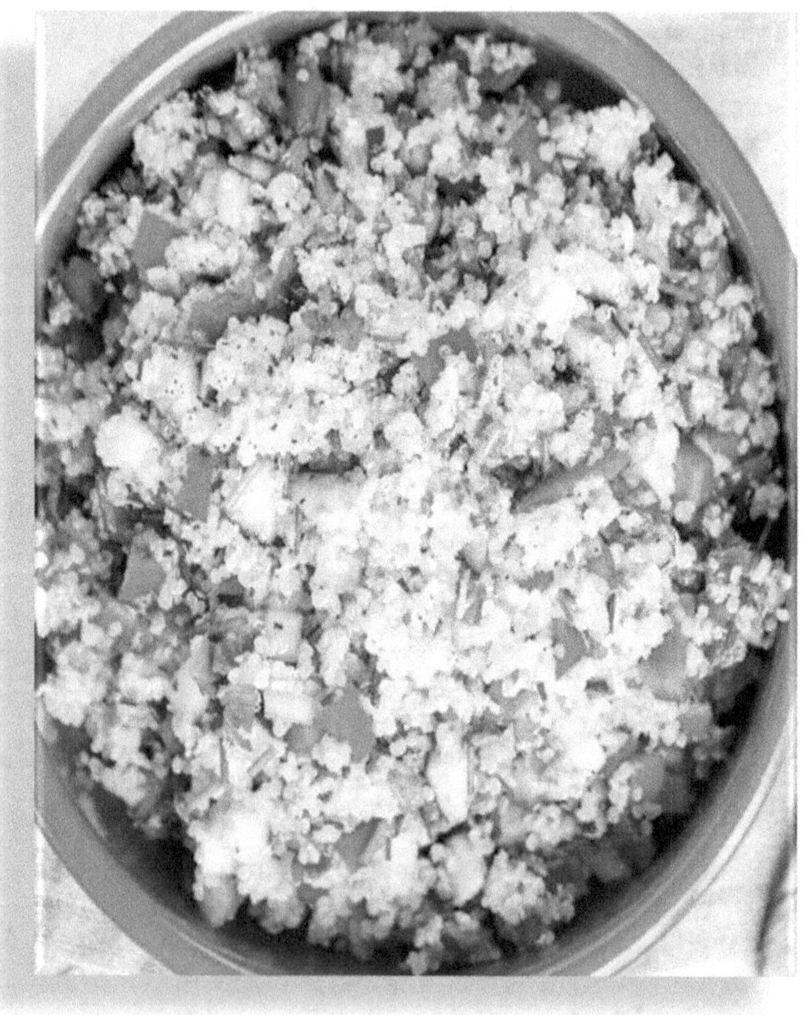

# Daily Affirmations for Individuals Facing Breast Cancer Challenges

1. "Discover your strength in moments when perseverance seems impossible."

2. "Each day is a new chapter in your journey; craft a narrative of resilience and optimism."

3. "Your path may be arduous, but always remember, you are resilient."

4. "In adversity, let your courage outshine your fears."

5. "Today's struggle becomes tomorrow's fortitude. Keep battling."

6. "On this journey, remember you're not alone; seek support and let love be your remedy."

7. "Celebrate small victories joyously; let them fuel your determination."

8. "Embrace uncertainty, for within it lies the chance for personal growth."

9. "Your scars narrate tales of survival and triumph; wear them with pride."

10. "Acknowledge progress, irrespective of its size; every step forward is a triumph."

11. "Hope is the rhythmic heartbeat of the soul; keep yours resilient."

12. "Adversity is the refining dust that polishes the jewels of heaven."

13. "Let your faith eclipse your fears."

14. "Your strength is your unique beauty; let it radiate, warrior."

15. "Believe in yourself and your limitless potential; an unstoppable force against any obstacle."

16. "Though the journey may be lengthy, the destination is well worth the effort. Keep moving forward."

17. "Cancer may have initiated the fight, but you will conclude it with courage and resilience."

18. "Transform pain into power, wounds into wisdom."

19. "Your identity isn't shaped by illness but by your enduring strength."

20. "Wake up with determination and sleep with the satisfaction of resilience."

21. "You are not a victim but a survivor; let your strength inspire others."

22. "Cancer is formidable, yet so are you. Keep pressing on."

23. "Your body is robust, your mind is indomitable, and your spirit is unyielding."

24. "Life is challenging, my dear, but so are you."

25. "Doubts today limit tomorrow's possibilities."

26. "Courage is the triumph over fear, not its absence."

27. "Your journey is exclusively yours, shaping a more robust, wiser version of yourself."

28. "Today's pain becomes tomorrow's strength; believe in the healing power of time."

29. "Climb mountains for the view, not for an audience."

30. "Be the person your future self-will proudly acknowledges."

31. "Find the silver lining in adversity; there's always something to be grateful for."

32. "True strength is revealed not in displays but in silent victories."

33. "Your attitude steers your path; maintain a positive course."

34. "Challenges are presented because you can overcome them. Face them with courage and grace."

35. "The true essence of living lies in rising after every fall, not in avoiding falls altogether."

36. "Your body is in recovery, your mind is evolving, and your spirit is ascending."

37. "You are a warrior; each day's battle enhances your strength."

38. "Believe in your inner magic; miracles transpire when least expected."

39. "Your journey attests to the potency of resilience; keep progressing."

40. "In challenging times, don't question 'Why me?' but declare, 'Try me.'"

41. "You are not alone; enveloped by love, strength, and infinite possibilities."

42. "You're not merely surviving; you're thriving in the face of adversity."

43. "The human spirit prevails over all challenges."

44. "Today's struggles sculpt tomorrow's fortitude; keep persevering."

45. "While not every day may be good, goodness can be found in every day."

46. "Make each day count, forgoing the mere counting of days."

47. "Defeat isn't in losing; it's in ceasing to try."

48. "Your journey, though demanding, is sculpting you into a masterpiece."

49. "Even the darkest night concludes, making way for a new dawn."

50. "Consider yourself a masterpiece in progress; embrace the ongoing process and trust the journey."

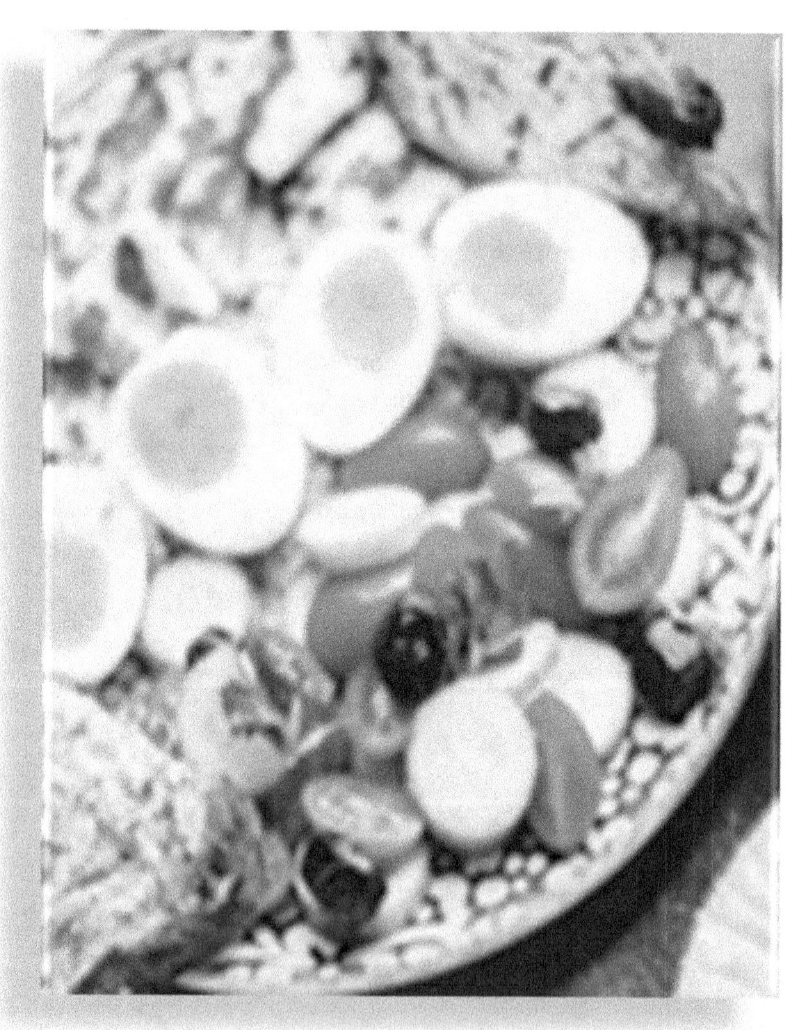

# CONCLUSION

In this Breast Cancer Diet Cookbook for Women over 50, A Culinary Companion for Seniors Navigating Breast Cancer" is not merely a cookbook; it is a heartfelt journey of nourishment, strength, and resilience tailored to the unique needs of our beloved seniors facing the challenges of breast cancer. Within these pages, we have embarked on a gastronomic odyssey, guided by the wisdom of age and the healing power of nutritious ingredients, all thoughtfully curated to support and uplift those on their cancer journey.

Through the artful combination of flavors and wholesome recipes, we have celebrated the joy of cooking and the comfort of familiar dishes, instilling a sense of hope and empowerment with each culinary creation. These pages have become a treasure trove, brimming with recipes designed to nourish not just the body but the soul, a testament to the profound connection between food and healing.

As we navigate the complexities of breast cancer, we recognize the profound importance of self-care and compassion. This cookbook serves as a warm companion, inspiring seniors to embrace their journey with grace and fortitude, while celebrating the rich tapestry of life through the aromas and tastes of lovingly prepared meals.

In the twilight of life, we find strength in the knowledge that small choices can make a profound difference. The meals we savor and share become a poignant reminder of our resilience, our capacity to find joy amidst adversity, and our unwavering determination to embrace every moment.

With this " Breast Cancer Diet Cookbook for Women over 50 " we honor the remarkable seniors who have shaped their lives, who now stand as beacons of courage and hope. Through these nourishing recipes, we celebrate the joy of connection, the power of community, and the triumph of the human spirit.

May each recipe within these pages be a testament to the love, care, and unwavering support of friends and family, walking alongside seniors on this journey. As the flavors intertwine, may they serve as a poignant reminder of the strength found within and the resolute determination to overcome life's challenges.

In closing, let us continue to cook, to love, and to treasure every moment, knowing that through the embrace of flavor, you nourish not just your bodies but the essence of life itself. To our seniors facing breast cancer, you are not alone. May these recipes serve as a culinary companion, reminding you that you are cherished, supported, and celebrated every step of the way. With hearts full of love and taste buds awakened, may we face the future together, in the warm embrace of flavors.

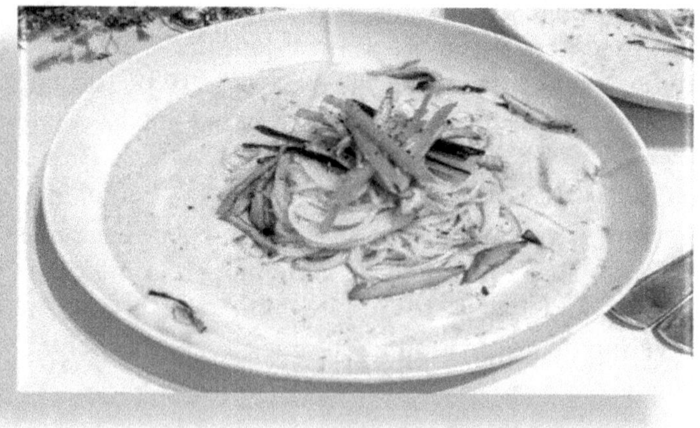

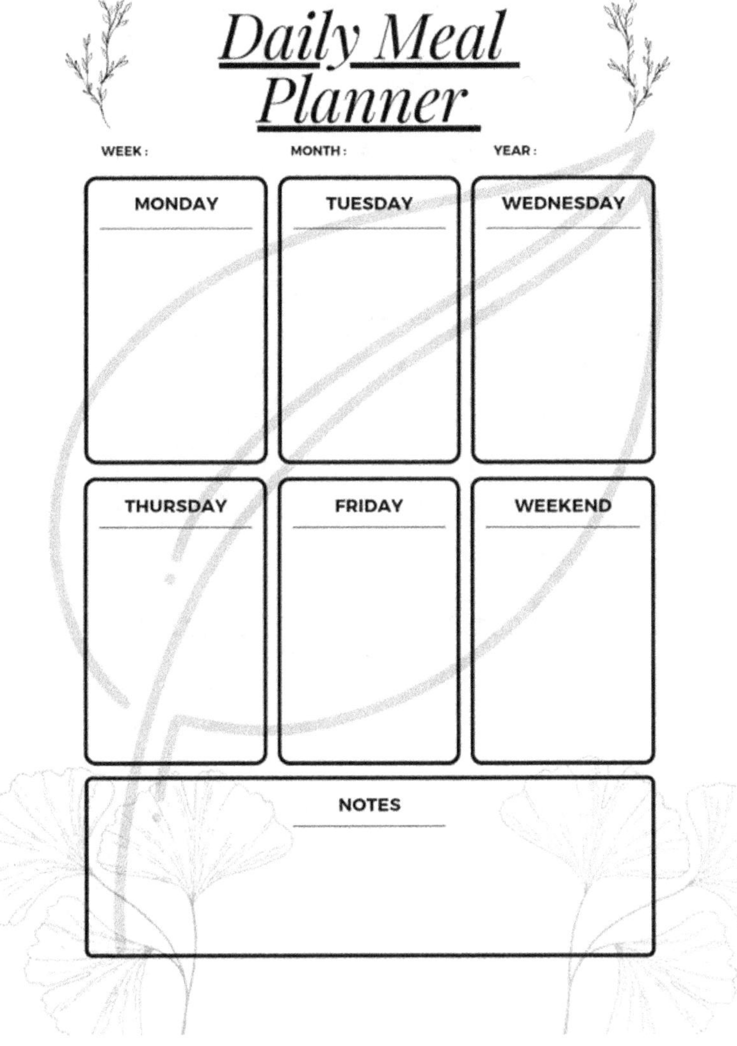


Daily Meal Planner

WEEK :

MONTH :

YEAR :

MONDAY

TUESDAY

WEDNESDAY

THURSDAY

FRIDAY

WEEKEND

NOTES

# Daily Meal Planner

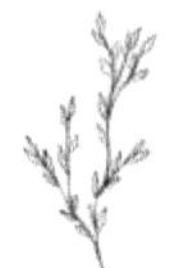
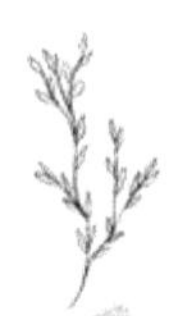

WEEK :  MONTH :  YEAR :

**MONDAY**

**TUESDAY**

**WEDNESDAY**

**THURSDAY**

**FRIDAY**

**WEEKEND**

**NOTES**

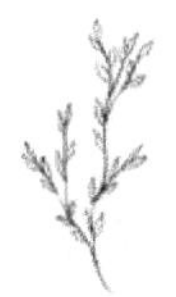 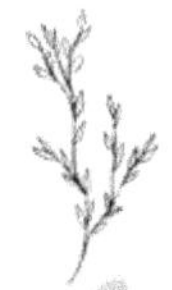

# *Daily Meal*
# *Planner*

WEEK :          MONTH :          YEAR :

| MONDAY | TUESDAY | WEDNESDAY |
|---|---|---|

| THURSDAY | FRIDAY | WEEKEND |
|---|---|---|

## NOTES

# Daily Meal Planner

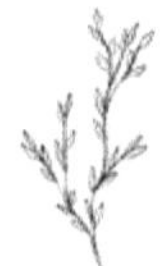
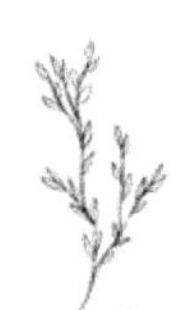

**WEEK :**  **MONTH :**  **YEAR :**

| MONDAY | TUESDAY | WEDNESDAY |
| --- | --- | --- |
| | | |

| THURSDAY | FRIDAY | WEEKEND |
| --- | --- | --- |
| | | |

**NOTES**

# Daily Meal Planner

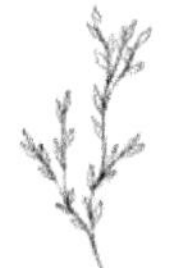
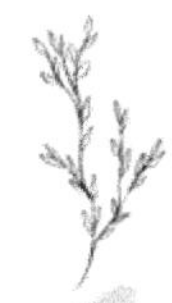

WEEK:        MONTH:        YEAR:

| MONDAY | TUESDAY | WEDNESDAY |
|---|---|---|
|  |  |  |

| THURSDAY | FRIDAY | WEEKEND |
|---|---|---|
|  |  |  |

**NOTES**

# *Daily Meal Planner*

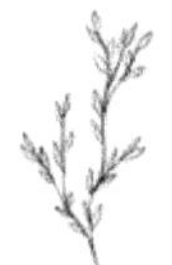
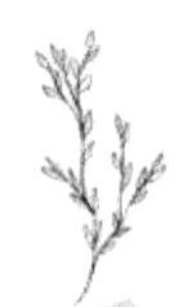

WEEK :          MONTH :          YEAR :

| MONDAY | TUESDAY | WEDNESDAY |
|---|---|---|
|  |  |  |

| THURSDAY | FRIDAY | WEEKEND |
|---|---|---|
|  |  |  |

**NOTES**

# *<u>Daily Meal Planner</u>*

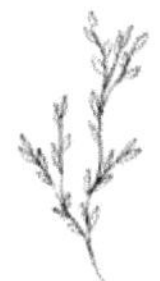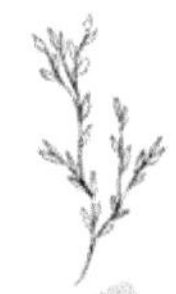

WEEK :  MONTH :  YEAR :

| MONDAY | TUESDAY | WEDNESDAY |
| --- | --- | --- |
| | | |

| THURSDAY | FRIDAY | WEEKEND |
| --- | --- | --- |
| | | |

**NOTES**

# Daily Meal Planner

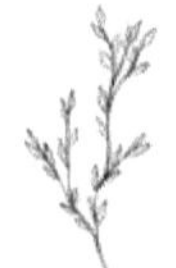
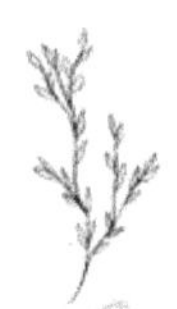

WEEK :          MONTH :          YEAR :

| MONDAY | TUESDAY | WEDNESDAY |
|---|---|---|
| | | |

| THURSDAY | FRIDAY | WEEKEND |
|---|---|---|
| | | |

### NOTES

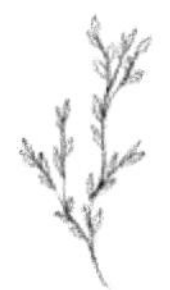
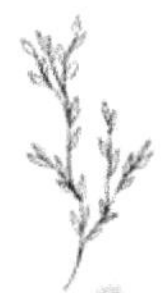

# *Daily Meal Planner*

WEEK :      MONTH :      YEAR :

| MONDAY | TUESDAY | WEDNESDAY |
| --- | --- | --- |
| | | |

| THURSDAY | FRIDAY | WEEKEND |
| --- | --- | --- |
| | | |

**NOTES**

# Daily Meal Planner

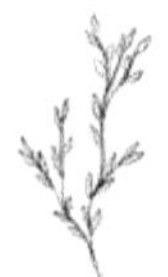 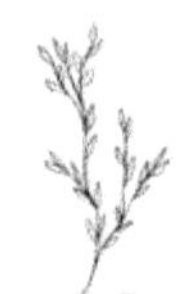

WEEK :          MONTH :          YEAR :

| MONDAY | TUESDAY | WEDNESDAY |
| --- | --- | --- |
|  |  |  |

| THURSDAY | FRIDAY | WEEKEND |
| --- | --- | --- |
|  |  |  |

NOTES

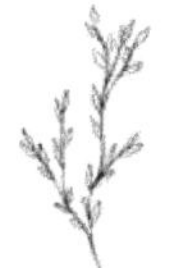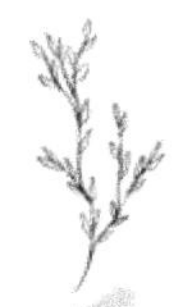

# *Daily Meal Planner*

WEEK :          MONTH :          YEAR :

### MONDAY

### TUESDAY

### WEDNESDAY

### THURSDAY

### FRIDAY

### WEEKEND

### NOTES

# *Daily Meal Planner*

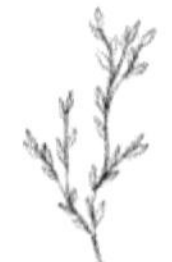
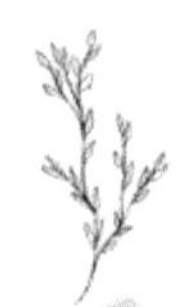

**WEEK :**   **MONTH :**   **YEAR :**

## MONDAY

## TUESDAY

## WEDNESDAY

## THURSDAY

## FRIDAY

## WEEKEND

## NOTES

# Daily Meal Planner

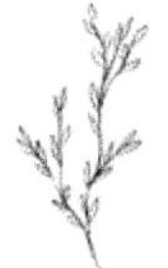 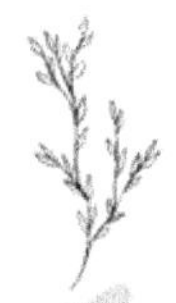

WEEK :          MONTH :          YEAR :

| MONDAY | TUESDAY | WEDNESDAY |
|---|---|---|
| | | |

| THURSDAY | FRIDAY | WEEKEND |
|---|---|---|
| | | |

**NOTES**

# Daily Meal Planner

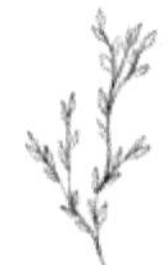 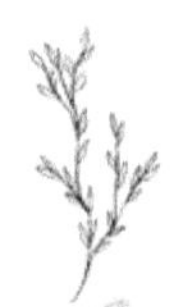

WEEK :    MONTH :    YEAR :

| MONDAY | TUESDAY | WEDNESDAY |
|---|---|---|
|  |  |  |

| THURSDAY | FRIDAY | WEEKEND |
|---|---|---|
|  |  |  |

**NOTES**

# *Daily Meal Planner*

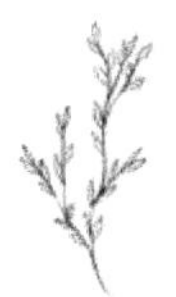
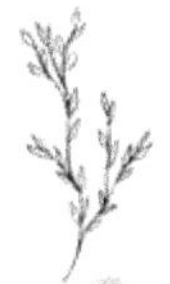

WEEK :  MONTH :  YEAR :

|  |  |  |
| --- | --- | --- |
| **MONDAY** | **TUESDAY** | **WEDNESDAY** |

|  |  |  |
| --- | --- | --- |
| **THURSDAY** | **FRIDAY** | **WEEKEND** |

**NOTES**

# Daily Meal Planner

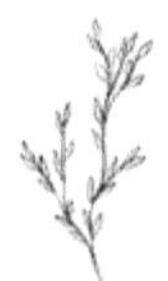 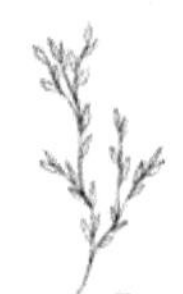

WEEK :          MONTH :          YEAR :

| MONDAY | TUESDAY | WEDNESDAY |
|---|---|---|
| | | |

| THURSDAY | FRIDAY | WEEKEND |
|---|---|---|
| | | |

## NOTES

# Daily Meal Planner

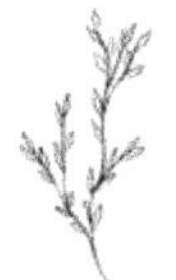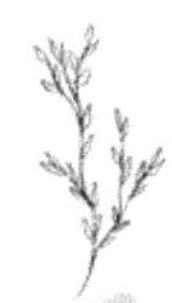

WEEK :          MONTH :          YEAR :

| MONDAY | TUESDAY | WEDNESDAY |
|--------|---------|-----------|
|        |         |           |

| THURSDAY | FRIDAY | WEEKEND |
|----------|--------|---------|
|          |        |         |

NOTES

# Daily Meal Planner

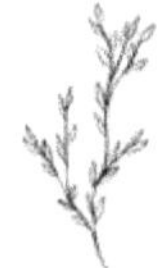
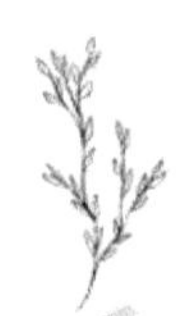

WEEK :   MONTH :   YEAR :

### MONDAY

### TUESDAY

### WEDNESDAY

### THURSDAY

### FRIDAY

### WEEKEND

### NOTES

# Daily Meal Planner

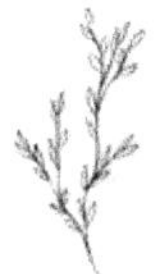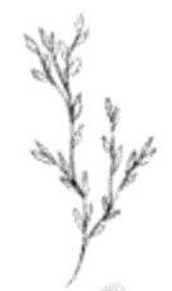

WEEK :  MONTH :  YEAR :

### MONDAY

### TUESDAY

### WEDNESDAY

### THURSDAY

### FRIDAY

### WEEKEND

### NOTES

# Daily Meal Planner

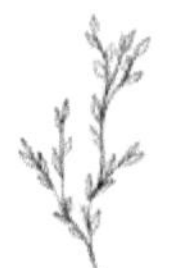
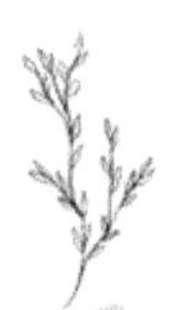

WEEK :          MONTH :          YEAR :

| MONDAY | TUESDAY | WEDNESDAY |
| --- | --- | --- |
|  |  |  |

| THURSDAY | FRIDAY | WEEKEND |
| --- | --- | --- |
|  |  |  |

## NOTES

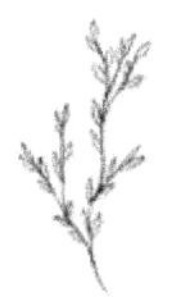 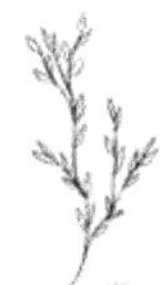

# *Daily Meal Planner*

WEEK :          MONTH :          YEAR :

| MONDAY | TUESDAY | WEDNESDAY |
| --- | --- | --- |
| | | |

| THURSDAY | FRIDAY | WEEKEND |
| --- | --- | --- |
| | | |

**NOTES**

# Daily Meal Planner

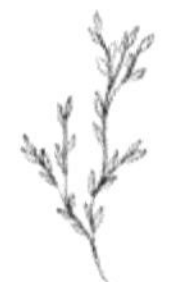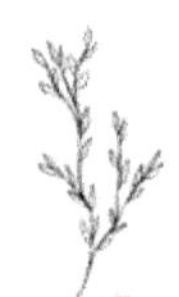

WEEK:      MONTH:      YEAR:

| MONDAY | TUESDAY | WEDNESDAY |
|---|---|---|
|  |  |  |

| THURSDAY | FRIDAY | WEEKEND |
|---|---|---|
|  |  |  |

## NOTES

# *Daily Meal Planner*

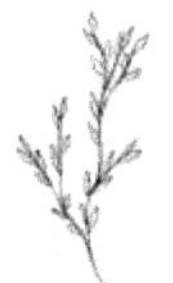 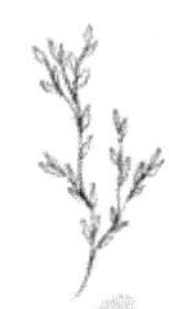

**WEEK :**  **MONTH :**  **YEAR :**

| MONDAY | TUESDAY | WEDNESDAY |
|---|---|---|
| | | |

| THURSDAY | FRIDAY | WEEKEND |
|---|---|---|
| | | |

**NOTES**

# Daily Meal Planner

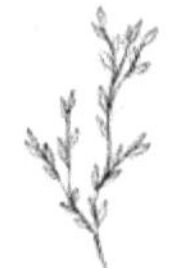
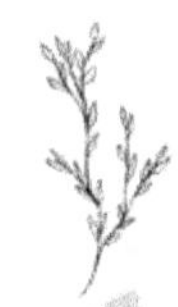

WEEK :  MONTH :  YEAR :

| MONDAY | TUESDAY | WEDNESDAY |
| --- | --- | --- |
| | | |

| THURSDAY | FRIDAY | WEEKEND |
| --- | --- | --- |
| | | |

## NOTES

# Daily Meal Planner

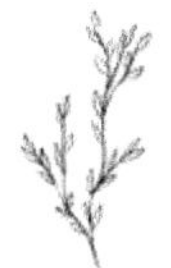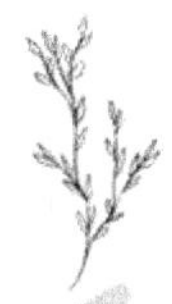

WEEK :          MONTH :          YEAR :

| MONDAY | TUESDAY | WEDNESDAY |
| --- | --- | --- |
|  |  |  |

| THURSDAY | FRIDAY | WEEKEND |
| --- | --- | --- |
|  |  |  |

## NOTES

# Daily Meal Planner

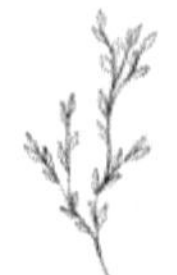
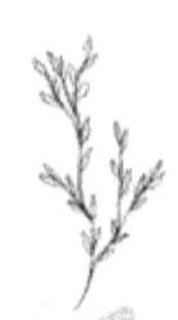

WEEK :          MONTH :          YEAR :

### MONDAY

### TUESDAY

### WEDNESDAY

### THURSDAY

### FRIDAY

### WEEKEND

### NOTES

# Daily Meal Planner

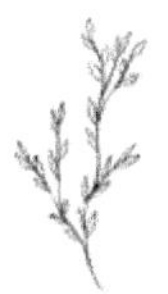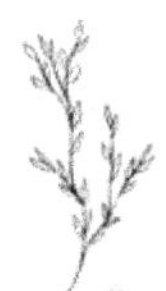

WEEK :          MONTH :          YEAR :

| MONDAY | TUESDAY | WEDNESDAY |
|---|---|---|
| | | |

| THURSDAY | FRIDAY | WEEKEND |
|---|---|---|
| | | |

## NOTES